# Moving a Relative with Memory Loss
## A Family Caregiver's Guide

Laurie White, M.S.W.
and
Beth Spencer, M.A., L.M.S.W.

first printing © 2000
second edition © 2006
Whisp Publications
P.O. Box 5426
Santa Rosa, CA 95402
www.whisppub.com

ISBN 0-9707609-1-4

Cover design and page layout by Jeff Reynolds Design

# Table of Contents

# Acknowledgments

We dedicate this book to all the family caregivers
with whom we have worked and from whom we
have learned. It is our hope that these pages –
the wisdom of many family members –
will help others in the future.

And to our own families – thanks for your
encouragement and support. Special thanks to
Brock Bowen and Erich L. Graf.

# INTRODUCTION

*Gail resisted all attempts by her kids to move her husband, Tom, to residential care. His memory loss and confusion had been increasing over the past two years, and Gail sometimes struggled to keep up with Tom's level of activity as he walked around the neighborhood, took things out of closets, and was up and down all night. She felt it was her job and her responsibility to keep Tom at home where he wanted to be.*

*When Gail had a heart attack and was in the hospital, her kids moved Tom to an assisted living residence that specialized in dementia care. Gail was not happy but understood that her kids all had jobs and couldn't provide care. When she got home and was back on her feet, Gail went to visit Tom with the intention of bringing him back home. Much to her surprise, Tom did not mention coming home. He proudly showed her around the residence where he had made friends and was actively involved in a number of activities. She realized that he had adjusted well and in many ways had a happier life than before.*

Not every person's move to residential care is as smooth as Tom's, but there are many things that family caregivers can do to ease the transition. This book has grown out of our many years' combined experience in working with family members who are caring for relatives with dementia. We know that moving a relative to residential care can be one of the most difficult decisions that family members will ever have to make. It is our hope that the ideas contained here will help families begin to think about some of the issues involved in moving, and will give them practical ideas for making this an easier process.

## About the authors

Laurie White, M.S.W., and Beth Spencer, M.A., L.M.S.W., have both worked with family caregivers in a variety of settings, including support groups, counseling, and residential care settings. Together, they owned a business in Ann Arbor, Michigan - *Caregiver Connection*, through which they offered counseling and care management services to older adults and training programs to family and professional caregivers. Laurie and Beth have conducted dementia training programs around the country and also are two of the co-authors of ***Understanding Difficult Behaviors***.

Laurie is a consultant and lecturer based in Santa Rosa, California. As owner of Dementia Care Consulting, Laurie provides counseling and care management services to families. She also consults with residential care homes on developing and expanding programs for families and direct care staff. Laurie has been affiliated with the Alzheimer's Association, both in Michigan and California, for nearly 25 years, most recently as Regional Director for the North Bay Area of the Alzheimer's Association of Northern California. Laurie lives in Santa Rosa, California.

As of this printing Beth is the Director of the Silver Club, a dementia adult day program associated with the University of Michigan's Turner Geriatric Clinic.

Prior to holding this position, Beth was Assistant Professor of Gerontology at Madonna University in Michigan, where she developed and coordinated an undergraduate certificate in dementia care. Beth is also co-author of ***Developing Meaningful Connections with People with Dementia: A Training Manual***, that has been used as an in-service guide throughout Michigan. Beth lives in Ann Arbor, Michigan.

## Some definitions

### Memory loss, confusion, dementia, Alzheimer's disease, etc.

In this book we are addressing the needs of people who have cognitive changes, such as memory loss, confusion, difficulty thinking clearly and making decisions, and possibly other symptoms. These problems are often called dementia, which simply is a word for a group of symptoms that can have many causes.

Some of your relatives may only have memory problems, some may have a diagnosis of Alzheimer's disease or a related illness; others may not have a diagnosis at all. Throughout these pages, we will use the terms memory loss, confusion, and dementia somewhat interchangeably. We are well aware, however, that there are many causes of and many individual variations with these types of symptoms.

Memory loss that interferes with normal day to day activities is not considered "normal" aging. Usually it is related to a disease process in the brain, although some people develop a condition called **mild cognitive impairment (MCI)**, which is limited to memory loss without other cognitive problems.

**Alzheimer's disease** is the most common cause of progressive dementia (dementia that gradually gets worse over time). There is enormous variation in the experience of individuals with Alzheimer's disease. The National Alzheimer's Association states the disease can last from 3-20 years; the average length of time is 8 years. There are over 70 identified causes of dementia. Other common causes are small strokes (also called **vascular dementia**, or multi-infarct dementia), **Diffuse Lewy Body Disease, frontal lobe dementias**, and many more.

If your relative has not had a good medical work up and diagnosis to determine the cause of the symptoms she is experiencing, we highly recommend

that you arrange to do this. There are some medications that may slow the progress of some of these disorders. Also, there are some treatable causes of dementia symptoms, which may be identified in a good diagnostic work up. Finding a diagnostic center or a physician with extensive experience in this field is helpful; your local chapter of the Alzheimer's Association, or the Area Agency on Aging can help you find clinics. (See *Locating Residential Care Homes* for information on finding resources.)

We also recommend that you contact your local chapter of the Alzheimer's Association to get more detailed information about dementia. We have included a reading list at the end of this book.

### Residential care homes, assisted living, nursing homes, etc.

Just as we are addressing this to the needs of individuals with a wide range of symptoms and diagnoses, we are also including a wide range of residential living situations. One of the difficulties is that the **names and licensing categories of residential care vary from state to state.** Assisted living is defined narrowly in some states, broadly in others. Small group homes may be called foster care or board and care homes. Nursing home levels of care and regulation vary from state to state, even though there are federal mandates for nursing homes. There are also different names for long term care facilities in different states: nursing homes, convalescent hospitals, etc. "Special care units" for people with memory loss or dementia are licensed and regulated in some states and not in others.

Because of this variation, in writing this book we are faced with a dilemma about what to call residential care. For the most part we have chosen not to use the term "facility" because it is a very institutional term. Some of the ideas we suggest may apply more to assisted living than nursing homes. However, most apply to a broad range of living situations.

For the most part, we have opted to use "residential care" or "care home" to describe this whole range of possibilities. We recognize, however, that nursing home care may be very different from life in a private pay assisted living facility or in a small board and care home.

Again, we suggest that you contact your county or city Department on Aging, Area Agency on Aging, or local chapter of the Alzheimer's Association for help in sorting out the terminology in your area and in determining what level of care is best suited to your relative.

### Staff representative

There is no universal term for the person who shows you around a residential care home or coordinates the process of moving in new residents. For purposes of simplicity, we have used "staff representative" to designate the person who is your initial contact with the residential care home. In reality, the person's title might be director of admissions, move-in coordinator or director of social services.

### A word about gender

Throughout these pages, we have mostly used "she" or "her" to refer to the person with memory loss or dementia. Obviously we know that some of your relatives are men! We chose to use the female pronouns simply because there are so many more older women than men.

### Legal authority

We have assumed throughout this book, that you or other family members have the legal authority to make decisions about moving your relative. The terminology and law differ slightly from state to state. If you are not clear about your legal status in this area, we suggest you talk with an attorney, or direct questions to the Area Agency on Aging, or your local chapter of the Alzheimer's Association.

### Case vignettes

We have included short case vignettes to illustrate how families have handled and reacted to various situations. While these are based on real situations, the names have been changed. These case studies are in the shaded green boxes throughout the book. We hope these case studies will help shed light on the range of situations and feelings that families experience in moving relatives.

### Individual experiences with moving

Your experience in moving your relative will depend on a number of different factors:

- Symptoms and difficulties your relative is having; where your relative is in the disease process.

- What kind of residential care setting you choose or can afford.

- The kind of relationship you have had with your relative in the past and present.

- Other stressful events happening in your life which may or may not be related to moving.

Obviously we are not able to account for all these factors in our general discussion and suggestions. We know that each family's experience with moving a relative with dementia is a unique one. We hope you will find some of our suggestions and examples helpful and will ignore the ones that don't pertain to your situation.

And lastly, read this book at your own pace. Some of you may find it helpful to read it from cover to cover. Some of you may want to read one section at a time and proceed to the next section as you need it.

*Laurie White*
*Beth Spencer*

# THE DECISION TO MOVE YOUR RELATIVE

# KEEPING YOUR RELATIVE AT HOME

Over the years we have noticed increasing numbers of families keeping relatives at home longer. In some cases families are able to maintain a relative at home until the end of her life, but this is rare. There are no rights or wrongs. What is possible and desirable for some families is impossible and/or undesirable in others.

In our experience there are several key factors at work here:

- Size of support network. Those who have large extended families or friendship networks available to help with care are more likely to be able to sustain the person at home longer.

- Financial resources. Frequently it is more expensive to maintain the person at home and may be impossible for many families.

- Behavior or medical issues of the person. Some individuals with dementia are much easier to care for than others. People who don't sleep well at night, who are highly agitated or who are medically fragile may be much more difficult to care for in a home setting.

The term "respite care" means "giving the caregiver a break." Respite care encompasses different kinds of services to help sustain people in a home setting including the following:

**Adult day programs.** Some programs specialize in care for people with memory loss; others are more general. Some adult day programs are "medical or health models" and include medical services as a key component; others are "social models" that emphasize stimulation and socialization. There is great variation in admission and discharge criteria, as well as hours of operation. Some programs are able to handle a wide variety of behaviors and can keep people into the later stages; others are more restricted. Some are in secured spaces; others are not. Also there is a wide range of cost arrangements from strictly private pay to sliding scales and subsidized programs. The types of clients who are participating, the kinds of activities that are offered and the training of staff are all important things to research. Some day programs are subsidized or have sliding fee scales; some are strictly private pay. Sometimes Veterans benefits, long term care insurance, or Medicaid (not Medicare) will pay all or part of the cost. The National Adult Day Services Association can provide you with a list of state associations and a list of questions to ask and things to look for during a site visit: www.nadsa.org or 1-800-558-5301.

**Home care.** There are also many kinds of home care arrangements - from national home care chains, to local organizations, to individuals who work as private caregivers. Things to consider include: cost, availability of backup arrangements, bonding and insurance, dementia experience, training of staff. Most home care is private pay, but as with day programs, there may be subsidies, long term care insurance or other help with payment in some cases.

**Out of home respite care.** This type of care is sometimes available in assisted living, small group homes or nursing home settings. Out of home respite is a temporary arrangement (usually depending on the availability of beds) where the individual with memory loss moves into a 24 hour setting for a specified period of time – ranging from a few days to a month. Families sometimes use this option when they are exhausted, when there is a family emergency or out of town event, or as a way to test out how their relative does in residential care. Different kinds of pay arrangements may be available depending on the setting and the geographic location.

Many times families who use a combination of respite services seem to be able to maintain their relatives at home for long periods of time. It can be helpful to use both day programs and home care. The day program gives the caregiver time alone at home and offers socialization and stimulation for the person with memory loss. Having a companion in the home allows the caregiver to get out and helps the family member with dementia get used to other people providing care and companionship. When care in the home or a day program is no longer viable, the transition to residential care may be easier. The same is true for people who have experienced out of home respite care - sometimes this eases the way to a permanent move to residential care for both the caregiver and the person with memory loss.

# MAKING THE
# DECISION TO MOVE

Some people in the early stages of memory loss recognize their need for more assistance with personal care and activities. However, most people with memory problems do not initiate a move or move voluntarily. Often, their insight into their own behavior and needs has been impaired. This is a common result of the brain damage caused by diseases such as Alzheimer's disease, small strokes, or similar illnesses.

Thus, it is usually the family of the person with memory problems who will recognize the need to move, find a place, and make the final decision to move.

Your decision of when your relative might move depends on your personal situation. Although there are no magic signs to tell you "this is the right time," many caregivers move their loved one to a residential care home for one or more of the following reasons:

*It is usually the family of the person with memory problems who will recognize the need to move, find a place, and make the final decision.*

- The amount of supervision and assistance needed by the relative with memory loss is too exhausting for the caregiver.

- Family members are not able to provide the necessary level of care due to family disagreements or geographic distances.

- The person with memory loss is no longer safe in her current residence.

- The caregiver is unable to keep up with both family and work responsibilities.

- Emergency and crisis situations for the caregiver or the person with memory loss have arisen.

- Illness or injury to the person with memory loss.

- The current level of services is not enough, is too expensive, or is too difficult to arrange and sustain.

- The person with memory loss no longer recognizes her home or family.

If you and your family are having one or more of these experiences, it may be time to start investigating other care options, including residential care homes. Even if none of these things is happening in your family, advance planning is recommended in order to give you the widest range of alternatives. Many families find that selecting a place gives them peace of mind, even though they may not need it for a long time. Of course, not all families are able to plan ahead for various reasons.

# ADVANTAGES AND DISADVANTAGES TO MOVING

Because this is such a hard decision, you may find it helpful to sort through the pros and cons of staying home versus moving your relative to residential care. We have listed below some of the common arguments we have heard and seen:

## Advantages of staying home

- My relative remains in a familiar environment.
- My relative doesn't want to move.
- Our family has more control over supervision and care.
- Our family feels they can provide superior care.
- Our family is honoring promises made.
- It may be less expensive.
- There is continued companionship for the caregiver.
- My family member enjoys caregiving.

## Disadvantages of staying home

- Providing 24 hour care can be exhausting, sometimes impossible.
- It may be too expensive to keep her at home.
- It can be very difficult to get adequate care at home.
- Our family may have too many competing demands, such as children, jobs, etc.
- No one in our family is available to provide or monitor the care.
- Our family may not be psychologically or

*Providing 24 hour care can be exhausting, sometimes impossible.*

physically able to cope with the demands of caregiving.

- My relative may have behavior problems that are too difficult to manage at home.
- The physical environment of our home may not be appropriate or safe for our relative in later stages.

## Advantages to moving to residential care

- By moving earlier in the disease process, my relative may be able to make friends with other residents and staff, enjoy activities, and adapt to the environment.
- There is 24 hour supervision available.
- Social and recreational activities are provided.
- My family can share the care with staff.
- The staff may be able to cope with some behaviors more easily.
- My relationship with my relative may improve since I am no longer providing care.

## Disadvantages to moving to residential care

- My relative is in an unfamiliar environment.
- The opportunity for doing some activities may not be present.
- They may not provide the standard of care that my family expects.
- The schedule or routines may not fit with that of my relative.
- My family may be uncomfortable with other residents.
- My relative may be more confused and disoriented during the initial weeks.
- My relative's mood may be affected by the relocation.

*You may find it helpful to write your own list of the advantages and disadvantages of each alternative. Writing this down sometimes helps clarify thinking.*

If you are struggling with this decision, you may find it helpful to write your own list of the advantages and disadvantages of each alternative. Writing this down sometimes helps clarify thinking.

# WHY MOVING IS HARD

*Harriet had been able to sustain her mother in an independent apartment by spending increasing amounts of time with her and hiring help from a home care agency. However, it was taking an increasing toll on Harriet, her husband, and her 3 young children. They considered moving her mom in with them, but she was terribly restless at their house and had walked out the front door and started down the street more than once. Finally Harriet realized she would have to move her mother. She carefully evaluated the options and the finances and made a decision. She had promised her mom she would never move her to a nursing home and now found that she had no choice. She said, "The day I moved my mom was the hardest day of my life."*

Over the years, we have heard stories like this one from family members. We want to acknowledge right up front that moving a relative into residential care is an extremely difficult emotional task. Sometimes families have doubts for many years about whether relocation was the right decision.

There are many reasons why moving a relative is so difficult. Some of the most common include:

**Media depictions of long term care.** Most of the time, what we see on TV or read in the paper is about the abuses in nursing homes or assisted living facilities. Many of our beliefs and fears are shaped by media images. It is a rare story that features the millions of caring, positive staff, the innovative programs, and the happy moments of life in residential care.

**Wedding vows** that include "in sickness and in health, 'til death do us part." Many spouses feel they are violating their marriage vows by moving their partner to residential care.

**The notion that** *"my mother cared for me, now it is my turn to care for her."* Raising children and caring for a parent with dementia are not

> **W**e want to acknowledge right up front that moving a relative into residential care is an extremely difficult emotional task.

7

equivalent, for many reasons, even though some of the tasks are similar.

**Old promises to parents, spouses or partners.** Unfortunately, we can never predict exactly what life will bring, and diseases such as Alzheimer's or small strokes are among the things that no one wants to think about. We may have made promises that we simply cannot keep.

**Family or friends who criticize.** Sometimes those around us reinforce the guilt and pain with insensitive comments, or with their beliefs (even though they are not the ones providing 24 hour care). You are the only one who knows what you can or cannot do.

**Moving symbolizes the decline of the person.** For many family members, the move to residential care is a very powerful symbol of the fact that the disease is progressing and the person is slipping away.

**Feelings of failure.** Many families feel their relative is getting worse because they have not tried hard enough. It is difficult to accept that many forms of dementia worsen over time, despite our best efforts.

Some things to keep in mind as you struggle with this difficult decision:

**You are not alone.** The majority of families find this one of the hardest, most painful decisions they have ever made.

**There are no clear rights and wrongs** when it comes to the care of a person with memory loss. If you weigh the pros and cons of various alternatives, you will probably find that there is no totally positive outcome. You may feel you are making the least negative choice of all your options.

**Know that your caregiving does not end at the door of the residential care setting.** You are still a caregiver, though your tasks may be different. Also, be aware that stress levels do not necessarily decrease with a move – you may find that you are still stressed, but the stresses are different.

**Keep in mind that your relative's adjustment may take months.** If you have moved in the past, you know that it can take a long time to adjust to a new place, new people, and giving up what you know and is familiar.

*It is difficult to accept that many forms of dementia worsen over time, despite our best efforts.*

Caregivers often say, *"No one can care for her as well as I have."* This is often true, and you will not find one-on-one care in residential settings. On the other hand, some people with memory loss actually function better and feel better in a setting with more people and activities, and when there are caring and consistent staff available.

There are things you can do to help yourself cope with the painful feelings that arise from this decision. We will talk about some of them throughout these pages.

# LOCATING RESIDENTIAL CARE HOMES

*After receiving a phone call from her mother's neighbor, Nancy realizes that her mother is no longer able to live in her apartment by herself. According to the neighbor, Nancy's mother, Mabel, has been hibernating in her apartment for several months. When she does come out she is not always able to find her way back without help. The neighbors are picking up groceries for her but much of the food remains in the refrigerator uneaten.*

*Nancy flies to see her mother and confirms the neighbor's concerns. Nancy tries to talk to her mother, but Mabel denies any problem and, in fact, becomes quite angry when Nancy talks about getting some help for her. Nancy returns home, knowing that she must find a place nearby where her mother can live safely. Where does she begin?*

**Where would you begin?** There are many available resources to get you started in locating a home, identifying the appropriate level of care, and give you the information and support that you may need.

Ask friends who may have moved a family member or know someone who has. Ask members of your local support group. Consult with your pastor, minister or rabbi.

Look in the yellow pages under:

- Alzheimer's Information and Referral Services
- Alzheimer's Care Facilities

- Assisted Living Facilities

- Residential Care Homes

- Nursing Homes

- Retirement and Life Care Communities and Homes

Contact your Employee Assistance Program (EAP) representative at work. Many corporations offer eldercare referral services.

Speak to the discharge planning or social service department, if your relative is in the hospital.

Look on-line. Many residential care homes have their own websites that describe their services and location(s).

We have listed websites and contact information for several organizations that offer general information about services for people with memory loss, including residential care. Many of the websites will link to additional related sites. This is a helpful resource list for families who are doing hands-on care, families who live close by or a long distance away. The information provided is current as of this printing.

***Alzheimer's Association.*** www.alz.org, 1-800-272-3900, 7 days a week, 24 hours a day.

The National Alzheimer's Association offers information about dementia and links you to local offices.

***Consumer Consortium on Assisted Living.*** www.ccal.org, (703) 533-8121, Monday-Friday

The Consumer Consortium provides materials to consumers on assisted living and advocates for residents' needs in assisted living settings.

***Eldercare Locator.*** www.eldercare.gov, 1-800-677-1116, 9 a.m.-8 p.m. EST, Monday-Friday.

Information specialists make referrals to state and/or local office on aging, who in turn, direct you to local resources.

***National Association of Professional Geriatric Care Managers.*** (NAPGCM) www. caremanager.org, (520) 881-8008, 8 a.m.-4:30 p.m. MST, Monday-Friday.

> *The National Alzheimer's Association's website offers you information about dementia, and also links you directly to local Chapters.*

NAPGCM helps locate care mangers, typically nurses or social workers, who assist families with care planning, health needs, moving, etc. Check with your local Area Agency on Aging or the Alzheimer's Association for care managers or placement specialists who are not affiliated with NAPGCM.

***National Citizens Coalition for Nursing Home Reform.*** www.nursinghomeaction.org, (202) 332-2275, 9 a.m.-5 p.m. EST, Monday-Friday.

National Citizens Coalition provides contact information for state and local Ombudsman offices and on federal and state regulations.

Try 'googling' the following titles:

- Assisted living facilities
- Nursing homes
- Senior housing
- Alzheimer's care
- Alzheimer's assisted living

Be aware that most referral sources will not make recommendations, though they may be able to help you narrow your search based on criteria such as the following:

- Geographic location
- Cost
- Long term care insurance, or Medicaid availability
- Level of service needed by your relative

Just learning the terminology in your state will be helpful. Your Area Agency on Aging or the Alzheimer's Association should be able to help you sort out some of these questions: Are you looking for a nursing home? Assisted living? Board and care home? A setting that is specially designed for people with memory problems or dementia? Or a more general setting for older adults?

# NEXT STEPS

**Phone screening.** Begin by calling the residential care homes you think will meet your needs. The answers you receive may determine whether you decide to visit or not. For example, if the cost of care is too expensive, you may decide not to visit and concentrate on the options available in your price range. Here are some questions to get you started:

- Do they accept people with memory loss? (Give as much information as possible about your relative's diagnosis and condition.)

- What is the monthly rate?

- What does the monthly rate include?

- Does the monthly rate change as a resident's care increases?

**Ask questions specific to your situation, such as:**

- Do they accept wheelchairs?

- Do they accept long term care insurance? Medicaid?

**Choose several places to visit.** If possible, choose places that will be convenient for you to visit once your relative lives there.

**Determine how many visits you can manage.** It can be quite emotional to talk with staff representatives about moving your relative. Try not to schedule too many visits in one day unless you are pressured to move your relative immediately.

**Call and schedule a visit.** Ask the staff representative to schedule a time for "talking and touring." Visiting during the most active times of the day for the residents will allow you to observe the residents and their interactions with staff. Ask how much time you should allow for the tour.

**Decide whether to include your relative in the selection of the residence.** Before you make this decision, visit several care residences. After you have chosen one or two, consider taking your relative to visit. Taking a person who is confused to visit unfamiliar places may be upsetting. See ***Visiting with (or without?) Your Relative***.

*Begin by calling the residential care homes you think will meet your needs.*

# PREPARING YOURSELF FOR THE VISIT

Feeling anxious or nervous is a common reaction for families who are getting ready to visit a care residence for persons with memory loss. Visiting may confirm that this is the right time to move a relative and brings the move a step closer to happening. It is understandable that this is an emotional time. It may help you to know what to expect during your visit:

- **Expect to feel a range of emotions.** It is not unusual to feel overwhelmed by the visiting experience, as well as by the range of feelings – relief, sadness, satisfaction, etc. The staff representative has likely seen many different family reactions to visiting and may be able to help you. If you feel overwhelmed, tell the staff member.

- **Be prepared to see residents with a range of abilities and needs.** Some residents may be more confused or physically frail than your relative while other residents may be less impaired.

*When Elizabeth visited Golden View she was shocked to see how frail and confused the residents were. Many were in wheelchairs, seemed unable to talk coherently, and were kind of frightening to her. Elizabeth could not imagine her grandmother in that setting with those people. Her friend pointed out to her, however, that all those people were somebody else's grandmothers and grandfathers – that other people saw them differently because they knew their life histories, who they had been and what they had done. Elizabeth realized that her own grandmother, at 90 years old with dementia, might appear to other families as confused and rather frightening.*

*It is not unusual to feel overwhelmed by the visiting experience, as well as by the range of feelings.*

- **Disruptions and unpredictable situations can occur.** Resident needs or emergencies may disrupt your visit. This is not uncommon during a family visit. If the staff representative needs to attend to a resident or a staff member, try to understand. Also be aware that even the best places have bad days. If you are not comfortable about what you are seeing, you may want to ask questions or visit again.

Before visiting residential care homes, it is important to know about government regulations, licensing and programs for staff and residents in different care settings. We have briefly discussed these topics below. Many of the resources listed in *"Locating Residential Care Homes"* can give you specific information on these topics as they pertain to assisted living, small group homes and nursing homes in your state.

**Paying for residential care.** The first thing to understand is that there are different kinds of residential care and each has its own payment structure. Nursing homes are usually financed differently from assisted living facilities which may be different from board and care homes. It is important that you find out the terminology and the payment structure in your state. The fact sheet on assisted living at www.eldercare.gov explains more about how finances work for assisted living.

Where your relative will end up living will depend to some extent on the financial situation. While there are some differences from state to state, generally it is important to understand the following:

- MediCARE does not pay for long term care for people with dementia. Medicare pays for hospital and rehabilitation care, but not for the long term day to day needs of people who have progressive memory loss. Medicare is a federal program.

- MediCAID is a combined state and federal program with some commonalities nationwide but many differences from state to state. Medicaid is for people who are low income and have used up most of their assets. Medicaid pays for a great deal of the nursing home care that is given to people with dementia who cannot afford nursing home rates privately. Although most assisted living care is paid for privately, in some states Medicaid may help with some of the costs. Consult with an attorney or expert so that you do not end up making poor choices about finances.

*There are different kinds of residential care and each has its own payment structure.*

**Licensing.** State licensing requirements vary; some types of residential care do not require licenses in some states. Nursing homes are heavily regulated; assisted living in some states is not. While this may give the care facilities more room for creativity, it also means that if there are problems, there is no agency to complain to. It is useful to know how licensing works in your state. Licensing agencies may be able to get you copies of inspection reports and complaints that have been registered. The resources listed on pages 10-11 should be able to help you find out more about licensing in your state.

**Ombudsman.** The federal government mandates that every state have a Long Term Care Ombudsman to act as an advocate for nursing home residents and their families. In some states, the Ombudsman also advocates for assisted living residents. The Ombudsman can provide you with information about complaints or problems with individual facilities that fall under their jurisdiction. To locate your state or local Ombudsman office, contact the National Citizens Coalition for Nursing Home Reform.

**Staffing.** An important factor to consider in evaluating the quality of care is the staffing level throughout the day. There is no universal staffing standard across the country for assisted living and small group homes. In nursing homes the federal government mandates that the staffing ratio be "adequate to care for the needs of the residents". However, the minimum staffing standard is determined by each state. The number of staff working with the number of residents is referred to as the staff to resident ratio. For example, 1:8 means 1 staff member is assigned to work with 8 residents.

**Staff Training.** In our experience, the most successful caregivers are those who are not only compassionate, caring, patient and flexible, but who have also received adequate training in caring for residents with memory loss. Staff who have had only a few hours of training about dementia care may not understand enough to provide the kind of care that you want. Again, dementia care training is not required in all care settings and states.

*State licensing requirements vary from state to state and in different types of residential care.*

**Activities.** Like all of us, people with memory loss have the need to do things that bring pleasure and meaning to their lives. A good activity program will offer activities to residents at all stages of memory loss throughout the day, alternating with restful periods. Activities are important as they can prevent boredom, depression, agitation or anxiety.

**The physical environment.** Many of the new assisted living facilities are beautifully designed and decorated. Sometimes families are so impressed by the physical appearance that they don't realize that the staff may not be well trained in dementia care or that the activity program is not designed for people with memory loss. Do not be sold solely on the basis of the physical plant. Also keep in mind what has appealed to your relative in the past. A woman with dementia recently said, "This place appeals to my daughter, but I've always liked simpler places. I don't like fancy hotels like my kids do."

On the other hand, individuals who have dementia are much more dependent on the physical environment for information and cues about how to behave and where to go than the rest of us. A well designed space with adequate lighting and signage, access to the outdoors, and interesting things in the environment can be extremely helpful and supportive to people with memory loss.

*Keep in mind what has appealed to your relative in the past.*

Additional questions to ask and things to look for during your visits are listed on the Worksheet for *Choosing a Residential Care Setting: Things to Look for, Questions to Ask* in the back of this book. By using this worksheet, you will be able to ask the same questions at each home and then have the needed information to compare residences on a variety of factors. This worksheet is intended to be copied.

# AFTER YOUR VISIT

Take a few minutes and reflect on your visit. Make further notes, if necessary about your overall impression of the staff, building, residents, etc.

**Ask yourself how you feel.** Jot down some words that describe how you felt being there: comfortable or uncomfortable, confident or unsure, attended to or neglected, etc. This exercise may give you a first impression that you can refer to later. Keep in mind that sometimes it is difficult to sort out your feelings about having to move your relative versus how you feel about the residence.

**Review your questions and answers.** Were all of your questions answered? Do you have additional questions to ask? If so, call the staff member who gave you the tour while the visit is fresh in your mind. Or schedule a return visit.

**Compare your list of questions and answers** with other places you have visited.

**Talk about your visit with other family members and friends.** Describe places you saw, things you liked, and your concerns.

**Visit more than once, if you have time.** Go at different times of day. You will see different staff and activities. Take other family members or friends with you, if possible.

# VISITING WITH (OR WITHOUT?) YOUR RELATIVE

*Gene has been caring for his wife Anne since her diagnosis of Alzheimer's disease five years ago. Gene has developed some health problems and realizes she needs more care than he can give. After Gene and his son James visited several care homes, they reserved a date and a room for Anne at Maple Lane. Although Gene has the legal authority to make this decision for his wife, he would like to talk to Anne about the move and take her to see her new room. James does not want to be the one to tell her and is concerned she won't move if she knows ahead of time. They agree they both want to do what is best for Anne, but how do they decide what that is?*

Making the decision to move a relative with dementia without involving her in the decision can be uncomfortable for families. For many caregivers it is the first time they have faced a major decision without consulting their spouse or parent.

The decision whether to take your relative to visit

before moving is a very individual one. Discuss visiting with or without your relative with the staff representative. She may be able to help you decide if a visit will benefit or be a drawback for your relative. However, be aware that some residential care homes may have never had a prospective resident with memory problems visit before moving in.

Here are some factors to consider:

**Your relative's needs and abilities.** Consider her ability to remember and understand as well as her ability to see, hear, and comfortably tour the building. Think about her reaction to seeing other residents.

**Extent of memory loss.** Some individuals' memory loss and disorientation are so extreme that a visit may not be worthwhile. On the other hand, you never know exactly which things your relative will remember or forget. (Often she may remember the very things you hope she will forget!) And even though she may not remember visiting by tomorrow, she may find the place familiar the next time she is there.

*By the time Marie's family made the decision to move her, she was nearly blind and severely confused. A visit beforehand would probably have increased her confusion and had few, if any, benefits.*

**Your family's ability to support her and each other simultaneously.** Some family members may be emotionally unavailable to support a relative with memory loss, due to their own emotional turmoil. If this is true in your family, you need to think carefully about your relative's needs during a visit. Who can spend time with her, reassure her and answer her questions?

**Past experiences and discussions.** It may help you to think about your relative's reaction to recent discussions or experiences with moving. They can be helpful in deciding whether to visit with your relative, but they are not always a good predictor of how she might react.

*Eve seemed quite willing to think about moving. She was a friendly former teacher, who seemed ideal for assisted living. She enjoyed her visit to the home, but on the day she actually moved, she created such a disturbance for a number of hours, that her family gave up and took her back home.*

*Joan, on the other hand, always told her kids, "The only way you'll get me out of my home is feet first." When she was taken for a visit to an assisted living facility, Joan raved about how lovely it was and began saying, "I'm moving here, and my kids can't stop me." She did move and adjusted well, in a short period of time.*

**The consequence.** Will she be more accepting or more resistant to moving? If she is more resistant, how will that affect your moving plans? How do you think visiting will affect her between the time you visit and moving day? Think about how your relative reacts if you tell her ahead about an important appointment. Does she forget about it? Does she stay up all night, agitated for two days? Is she more anxious but able to cope?

**Possible benefits** of visiting with your relative:

- It involves her in an important life decision.

- Visiting acquaints her with the environment and staff.

- You can observe her reaction to staff and residents.

- It may help relieve your guilt, especially if she is involved in the choice of places.

**Possible drawbacks** to visiting with your relative:

- It may increase her agitation.

- She may have a negative reaction to the environment and staff.

- It may increase her confusion.

- It may increase or cause paranoia or suspicion.

- She may not remember the visit. (But keep in mind that you will never know for sure what she does or doesn't remember.)

## On Your Visit Together

If you decide to introduce your relative to the care home before moving day, the following suggestions may help you:

**Inform the staff representative ahead of time.** Explain what you have told your relative about the visit. For example, if you tell your relative that you are going to visit a place you have heard about, you do not want the representative to say, "Oh, we are so glad you will be coming here to live." Tell the representative what might be comforting and upsetting for your relative to hear or see.

**Plan your visit around a meal or activity.** It is often helpful to include a pleasurable activity in the visit, such as a meal or an activity that you are sure your relative will enjoy. This takes advance planning with the staff.

**Keep the visit short.** The length of your visit should not exceed your relative's tolerance for being in an unfamiliar place. Watch for signs that may indicate she is ready to leave, such as a change in behavior or increased agitation.

**Observe your relative's reaction to caregivers and residents.** Watch body language and facial expressions. Does your relative seem to be concerned? Anxious? Scared? Pleased? How does she react to other residents? Does she have questions that you or the staff member need to answer? How are staff interacting with your relative? This may give you important information about the residence.

*It is often helpful to include a pleasurable activity in your visit.*

> *When Joyce took her husband Elmer to visit The Rose Garden Home, she was concerned that he would be angry. As they toured the building, Joyce noticed that Elmer was very interested in the residents and the activities that they were doing. He seemed relaxed as long as she was close by. Joyce felt reassured that Elmer could make friends here.*

# MAKING
# THE MOVE

# TALKING TO YOUR RELATIVE ABOUT THE MOVE

Some families find it difficult to talk to their relative with dementia about the approaching move. We believe that it is important to prepare your relative for this event, keeping in mind her unique needs and characteristics. You may feel unsure how and when to bring up the subject of moving, and who should be present for the moving discussion. We've listed below some things for you to think about.

**Decide when to tell your relative about the move.** "How far ahead of time should I tell my relative about the move?" There is no right or wrong answer to this question. When families tell their relative about the move depends on many factors including a loved one's ability to understand and cope with a pending move. Try thinking about past experiences when you talked about an event ahead of time. Did it cause unnecessary anxiety or did it help prepare her for the event? Some families find that telling their relative 24-48 hours ahead of time prepares their relative and themselves for the move. Other families wait until the day of the move because they are unsure how their relative will respond and how they will cope if their relative is resistant to moving.

*How far ahead of time should I tell my relative about the move?*

*When Mary was deciding when to tell her mother about the move, she remembered how anxious her mother became when she was told about a doctor's appointment ahead of time. Mary decided to take her mother to visit the residential care home on the scheduled move-in date and then tell her she would be staying there.*

*Delores told her husband that she was no longer able to care for him at home. She explained that she had found a nice place for him and she needed his help in getting ready. Over the next couple of days they worked together deciding what things he would take with him.*

**Decide who will tell your relative about the move.**
Who is the best person to tell your relative that she is
moving? It may be a family member, friend or
doctor. Generally speaking, the person talking with
your relative about the move should be someone
your relative knows and respects. Some families find
it is better to have more than one person present
when the idea of moving is brought up. Other
families find it is better for their relative to have only
one person there.

*Joe's family got together and decided that Virginia,
the oldest daughter, was the person who should talk
about the move with Joe because they had the closest
relationship.*

*No one in Sue's family wanted to talk to her about
moving. They asked Dr. Jones to get them started and
then they were able to talk to her openly. When Sue
would ask "Why do I have to move?" her family
would say, "It was Dr. Jones' recommendation."*

**Plan what you are going to say ahead of time.** It
may help to write it out or rehearse it with your
family or a friend. Think about how your relative
might react and prepare what you will say in answer
to her questions or concerns.

*John was nervous about telling his mother they had
reserved a room for her at the Alzheimer's unit. He
didn't know what to say. He practiced what he was
going to say with his cousin and felt more prepared
and confident when the time came to tell her.*

**Keep it simple and consistent.** For someone with
memory loss, a short, simple and consistent
discussion is usually the best. Details can be
confusing for some people. If your relative asks
questions about the move, be consistent in your
response. Use the same words in every answer. This
can be comforting to her and may help her
remember.

*The person
talking with your
relative about the
move should be
someone your
relative knows and
respects.*

*Ruth had Alzheimer's disease and would talk about her memory not working. When her sons talked to Ruth about moving, they said "Dr. Peters has made a reservation for you to stay at Charter House. He thinks they will be able to help you with your memory there. We will be taking you there on Friday."*

**Prepare an explanation that will be understood and accepted.** As you think about how to explain the reason for the move, it may help to think about past experiences that were enjoyed by your relative.

*Before she retired, Sonia often traveled for her job and it was not unusual for Edward to stay at a hotel while he accompanied her on the business trip. When it came time to move her husband, Sonia told him he would stay at the "inn" while she was on a business trip. He seemed to understand and was content to stay there when she left on the first day.*

**Is this deceitful?** The above case study brings up the issue of how honest and direct a family should be in talking about the reason a relative is moving. Some families are comfortable telling a person with memory loss a partial truth if it makes their relative feel better. Some families are not. The decision of what to say is a very individual one. Sonia felt that her explanation made sense to Edward and brought him comfort.

**Acknowledge her feelings.** If your relative expresses resistance, sadness, anger or other feelings, it is important to set aside the time to listen and offer reassurance. Acknowledging sad or angry feelings can be comforting to both of you. Too often, the feelings of people with dementia are ignored or discounted.

**Expect a change in mood and behavior.** Although this doesn't always happen, sometimes a person with memory loss can become more confused and agitated when a move is imminent.

*When Mildred's family could no longer care for their mother in their home, they talked about it openly with her. She understood and said she did not want to be a burden to them. Between the time that they talked and the actual move, Mildred packed and unpacked the suitcase dozens of times and repeatedly asked, "When are we leaving?"*

## If you decide not to tell your relative ahead of moving day:

**Realize you may behave and talk differently.** Even though you are trying not to, you may be showing tension, guilt, or other feelings. People with dementia are often very sensitive to other people's feelings even when they can no longer put names to them.

> *Caroline's family decided not to tell her about moving until the day of the move. They were very careful not to talk about the move in front of her but when they told her she said, "I know."*

**Plan what you are going to say if she asks.** Even if it is unlikely that your relative will ask what is happening, it is a good idea to have an answer ready.

> *Although Bill's family decided not to tell him about the scheduled move, they felt they needed to be prepared in case he asked. Bill's children all agreed to say, "The doctor thinks mom needs a vacation. While she is away, you will be staying at a place where they have great food and activities to do."*

**Watch for any changes in your relative's mood or behavior.** It is not unusual for a person with memory loss to react to your own anxiety or fatigue with agitation.

**Be prepared for strong emotional reactions when the move occurs.** If your relative really is surprised and unaware, it may be a shock. If this occurs, rely on the care staff to help you. There is a possibility that your relative may not react strongly to her new surroundings. When a new resident feels secure with the people and place, she may be more accepting than the family expects.

*Even though you are trying not to, you may be showing tension, guilt, or other feelings.*

# PLANNING FOR MOVING DAY

*Mabel did not want to move. Her daughter, Nancy, tried several times to talk to her mother about where she was moving but each time it was as if they had not talked about it before. Nancy decided to concentrate on what she could do to make the move as easy as possible for herself and her mother. Nancy thought that having all of her mother's possessions in place when she arrived would be welcoming and comforting. While Nancy took her mother to lunch, Nancy's sister decorated and furnished the room with their mother's belongings. When Mabel arrived, she was delighted to see her furniture, pictures on the wall, and her quilt on her bed.*

Your relative may or may not be as receptive as Mabel was to seeing her belongings in a strange place. This is one of the many things to think about as you plan for moving day.

Some families find it helpful to keep busy preparing for the move. Other families do not have the time or the energy to have everything completed before the scheduled moving day. To avoid feeling overwhelmed about the details of moving, divide the task list into three segments, before, during and after the move. The staff representative can help you decide what is important to do ahead of time and what things can wait until after your relative has moved in.

Here are some things for you to consider as you plan your time:

**Try to do some of the paperwork ahead of time, if possible.** Many care residences will encourage you to fill out the necessary forms ahead of time rather than on moving day. This allows you to be with your relative as she arrives at the care home, and is introduced to the staff and her room. If it is necessary for you to do the paperwork on moving day, ask how much time it will take, and what your relative will be doing while you complete the forms.

**Ask someone to help you on moving day.**
Although the residence's staff will help you and your relative get settled, it can be comforting for you and

*A**sk someone to help you on moving day.**

your relative to have someone familiar with you. A friend or a family member can offer you emotional support and give attention to your relative as you go through the move-in process.

*Mary was unprepared for how overwhelmed and sad she felt on the day they moved her mother. She was so glad that her friend, Gladys, had offered to come along. Gladys was able to chat with Mary's mother, answer her questions, walk around with her, and generally engage her. Mary had all she could do to handle the arrangements and cope with her own feelings.*

**Plan what to do after you leave your relative at her new residence.** It can be very helpful to take time for yourself as you transition into a new era of caregiving. You have spent a great deal of time and energy caring for her and planning this move. Plan to do something you would enjoy, such as a bath, dinner with a friend, a walk, etc.

*Sally had to be at work the day her mom moved her dad into the assisted living facility. Her mother wanted to go home in the evening when she left the care residence, so Sally went to her mother's house with some flowers and her favorite casserole and stayed with her mother for several hours. Although her mother had said not to bother, she was grateful for the company and the attention.*

**Think about what personal possessions you will move.** Many care residences encourage the family to bring personal items. Think about what items have special meaning to your relative. Some suggested items: a favorite chair, books, mementos, special awards, etc. Check with the staff representative about what residents are allowed to have and what might fit into the room or apartment.

**Put together a photo album or a wall collage of your relative.** A photo album or collage is not only a nice way for you to document your relative's life, but also can provide the staff with things to talk about with her. Include photos which show her interests, hobbies, family, and career. Label each photograph with dates, location and people's names. For example, "Joe stationed in England, 1943."

**Ask about decorating the room.** You can do this before or after your relative arrives. Personalizing the entrance to her room with decorations such as flowers, art work, or a wreath can feel very welcoming. It may also comfort her to enter a room already decorated with her favorite things such as photographs, a chair, and her afghan on her bed.

*Al felt too overwhelmed by the idea of moving to select items for his wife to take with her the day she moved to the care residence. After she moved in, he enjoyed taking items to her each time he visited. They both enjoyed talking about the things that he brought and decorating the room together.*

**Give the staff information about your relative.** Many residences have a "personal profile" form that lists a resident's past interests and accomplishments, her current routine, etc. This information can help the staff learn about your relative and feel more comfortable conversing and caring for her, which in turn can help your relative adjust to her new home and staff. If the care residence does not have a form, make a list of "Important Things to Know About My Relative." You can do this before or after your relative moves in.

**Consider how to help your relative feel most relaxed on moving day.** Following her daily routine on moving day may cause less confusion and fatigue. On the other hand, changing the routine by getting her hair done or going out to lunch on the way to the care home may help her feel special and relaxed.

**Plan the move at your relative's best time of day.** Check with the residence about the preferred time for moving. Try to match your relative's best time of day with their schedule. Things to consider: When does she feel most rested? When is she at her best physically? Is she in a better mood at a certain time of the day?

**Dedicate the entire day to moving.** Although the physical move-in may not take all day, families often feel the emotional and mental fatigue of the move. If possible, do not schedule other appointments on this day. After you have moved your relative, spend the rest of the day caring for yourself.

**Be aware that planning your relative's move can be quite emotional.** You may experience mood swings

*Make a list of "Important Things to Know About My Relative." You can do this before or after your relative moves in.*

from relief to doubt about your decision and be more fatigued than usual. These are normal feelings.

# MOVING IN

The feelings you experienced during the planning period may be more intense on moving day. Feelings of sadness, anxiety, and guilt are normal and even expected. Some families do not feel the full emotional impact of moving a loved one until moving day. Knowing this ahead of time may help you.

**Recognize that the best prepared plans might go astray.** Despite your best efforts, it is not always possible to follow a schedule or a plan for a person who is confused and forgetful. For example, you may arrive later than expected because your relative was particularly slow getting started in the morning. Try to be flexible and remain calm if things are not going as planned.

**Introduce yourself to staff.** These are going to be important people in the life of your relative and perhaps in your life, as well. Start off on a good foot with staff, even if everything is not perfectly to your liking.

**Depend on the staff to help you and your relative.** Let staff know if you are having a hard time or need some help. They are used to helping families with various aspects and feelings of moving.

**Ask for privacy if you need it.** If you need some time by yourself or with your relative, ask the staff where you might go for privacy in the building. This is a very common request and staff are usually very understanding and accommodating.

*As Hannah was putting her mother's things away in her closets and drawers, she became tearful. She was very appreciative when the move-in coordinator asked if she would like to go to the family room for some privacy. After a few minutes by herself, she was able to return to her mother's room and continue moving in her mother's clothing and personal items.*

**Tell the staff how to answer your relative's questions or concerns.** Let the staff representative know what you have told your relative about staying or living at the care residence. Ask the staff

*Making the Move*

*Some families do not feel the full emotional impact of moving a loved one until moving day.*

representative to notify all appropriate staff members how to answer expected questions. Consistency may help your relative's adjustment and reduce feelings of insecurity. Having the following items written out on a piece of paper can be an easy reference for staff:

- What you call her new home (apartment, hotel, name of residence, a place to help people with memory problems, etc.)

- How long she thinks she will be there (for awhile, several days, until she feels better, up to her doctor, etc.)

- The reason she is there (to help her with her memory, because she needs more help, per doctor's orders, etc.)

- What to tell her if she asks for you or other family members.

- What things not to say, things that will upset her (This is your home now., You are going to be living here now., This is a nursing home., etc.)

**Plan your visiting schedule.** If possible, before you leave, tell staff when you will be back to visit. Try to schedule your first visit within a few days after the move, unless otherwise recommended. Your visits are important because they allow you to learn the routine and develop relationships with staff. Visits can reduce feelings of abandonment for your relative.

**Ask for assistance with your departure.** It is very common to be concerned about how to leave your relative on the first day. This is especially true if you anticipate your relative will be angry or determined to go with you. Staff can be quite creative in supporting the new resident and the family when it is time for the family to leave and the resident to stay.

*It is very common to be concerned about how to leave your relative on the first day.*

> As Melanie was preparing to leave, Marvin insisted on going with her. No amount of explanation or reassurance seemed to help. A staff member asked Melanie and Marvin to join her for a cup of coffee. The staff person engaged Marvin in conversation and as Marvin began to relax, Melanie excused herself saying she "would be back shortly," and left for the day.

**Ask whom you should call for an update.** Find out who is assigned to your relative on each shift. Ask the staff representative whom to call if you want an update on how your relative is doing during the first few days.

# AFTER
# THE MOVE

# BUILDING RELATIONSHIPS WITH STAFF

The success of residential care is totally dependent on good staff. One way families can help themselves and their relatives is to develop relationships with staff members.

**Introduce yourself to all the staff.** "I am Frances' daughter. My name is Marsha and I will be visiting her during the week. My brother Dick will be visiting on the weekend." Sometimes staff are not good at introducing themselves, or may not be comfortable with families. The more you reach out, the better relationships you will develop. This will help you be better informed about your relative's progress and activities.

**Call staff by their names.** Addressing a staff member by her name is a good start to building a friendly and trusting relationship. Using a staff member's name can also prompt her to remember you and use your name when you visit.

**Pick your issues and know the complaint process.** It is terribly difficult to be a family member when things aren't going right. Families worry about complaining too much, about reprisals against their relatives, about nothing being done. It is important to know which staff members to go to for what, and to know the complaint process. It often works best to express your expectations rather than list your complaints.

**Give praise, too!** Don't forget to let staff know when you are pleased, when things are going right.

**Keep in mind that every residence has bad days.** There may be times when you are unhappy about the care your relative is receiving, or the state of her room or bathroom. Know that there will be days when unforeseen circumstances occur, such as short staffing. Try not to take it out on those who are there.

**Give staff time to get to know your relative.** And think about how to help. What do you want them to know about her? What are the pieces of

*Addressing a staff member by her name is a good start to building a friendly and trusting relationship.*

information that will make her come alive as a person with a history? What will help staff attend to her personal care?

> *Lynn worked hard to help staff get to know her sister. First, she created a photo collage that included labeled pictures of her sister throughout her life. Next she wrote a short biography of her sister's life, so that staff would know key events and important people in her life. Finally, Lynn tried to convey a little of what her sister had been like by writing down a few stories that illustrated important characteristics. For example, she described her sister's love of animals by talking about her pets and the volunteer work she had done at the Humane Society, including bringing home many strays. She also discussed the fact that her sister had always had a quick temper and did not tolerate frustration easily. To illustrate this, Lynn described her sister's attempts to learn to play the piano, when she would curse and pound on the keys in anger. Lynn felt it was important for them to know that there were lifelong traits that continued even after her dementia diagnosis.*

**Get involved in family activities.** Many residences have family education or support groups, and social events that include families. It may be helpful for you to become involved. You will learn more about how things work and will have a chance to get to know other families.

**Be a volunteer.** Most homes rely to some extent on volunteers to help with many kinds of activities and special events. This is another way to get to know staff, to be privy to what is happening, and to be involved in doing activities with your relative.

# SOME SUGGESTIONS FOR VISITING

Visiting your relative after she moves may raise many questions for you. Below are some suggestions for making visits easier.

**Plan your visiting schedule.** Some families find it helpful to have a regular schedule for visiting. This is often valuable for your relative as well, because it can be put on a calendar, or staff can be alerted to tell your relative the next time you will be there. However, when people are very confused and disoriented, they cannot always keep track of schedules. You will need to determine whether this will be helpful or more confusing for your relative.

**If you are concerned, call ahead** and ask if this is a good time and day to visit. Most care homes have fairly open visiting policies, although this will depend on what kind of residence your relative is in.

**Visit during different shifts, if possible.** You will see different staff and different activities.

## First visits:

**Plan what time to visit.** Ask the staff about visiting hours. If there are activities that she will be attending, ask if you can join her in the activity. Sometimes care residences will ask you not to visit initially during activities so your relative can develop relationships with other residents. Ask the staff for general guidelines of how often to visit during the first few days and weeks. Your visits are important as they confirm she will still see you even though she is living in a new place.

Some places have policies suggesting that families not visit for some period of time following the move (two weeks, one month, etc.), in order to allow the resident time to adjust. In our experience, this can be extremely devastating to the person with memory loss, making her feel abandoned, frightened, or hopeless. Question such a policy carefully.

**Be prepared!** Most of us, when we think of visiting, think of talking. But this is not always easy or possible with relatives who have memory loss and may have communication difficulties. Planning a simple activity such as a special snack, looking at magazines or photographs, or reading a letter together can help you feel more relaxed when you visit. And it can relieve you of the burden of making conversation. At the end of this section is a list of simple visiting ideas.

*Your visits are important as they confirm she will still see you even though she is living in a new place.*

*Max dreaded visiting his wife, as she no longer was able to stay focused on conversation. She seemed to have lost interest in news about the family and the neighborhood. Picking up on suggestions from staff, he began keeping a bag in the car with things that might interest Matilda. Some days he would take out several of the framed photos that had been in their den at home for many years. Other days, he played one of several tapes of hymns. Periodically he changed the objects in the bag, adding cookies and a nice plate to serve them on, taking out a book she had tired of. With a little planning, Max found visiting much easier.*

**Keep your visits short.** Remember that your relative may tire easily, that her attention span is probably limited, and that she very likely does not have an accurate concept of time – either how long you have been there or how long it has been since your last visit. Fatigue, agitation, and change of mood may be signs to end your visit.

**Keep your numbers down.** It can be overwhelming for some residents with dementia to have too many visitors at once. Be sensitive to what works for your relative. Perhaps on her birthday, she will do better with short visits from several groups, rather than a large family gathering.

**Responding to other residents.** Sometimes families are uncomfortable with the behavior of other residents. If you have questions or concerns, ask a staff member. Staff should be able to give you tips on how to respond to residents who may seem confused, insistent or upset. As you spend more time there, chances are you will develop friendly relationships with many of the other residents.

**Remember that the feelings inspired by your visits are more important than the content.** Conversation can be difficult sometimes. You may come with an activity in mind that does not seem to work at all that day. The most important goal of visiting is to share a pleasant moment (even though your relative may not remember it). Don't correct her or expect detailed answers to questions.

*The most important goal of visiting is to share a pleasant moment.*

*Doris enjoyed taking her mother out for snacks at a park by the river near the care home. Her mother always thoroughly enjoyed sitting at a picnic table eating the snack, which Doris laid out on a table cloth with cloth napkins and silverware. After they packed up and put things away, her mother would often say, "Oh, it would be nice to have a snack here someday." At first Doris was very upset that her mother did not remember the snack they had just eaten. But gradually she learned that even though the memory faded, the pleasant emotions stayed with her mother for hours.*

## Simple visiting ideas

**Visit during mealtime.** This gives you an opportunity to socialize with other residents, to see how mealtimes are handled and how your relative is eating.

**Visit during an activity of interest.** Check the activity schedule and go with your relative to an activity. This may help her become more involved and will give you something to do together.

**Bring some "props" from home**, such as a favorite food, a picnic, a photo album, a picture book that will interest your relative, simple poems or short stories to read together, a simple sewing or woodworking project, cards to write to relatives or friends, music, simple games.

**Learn to modify activities** to allow your relative to be successfully involved.

*At first Eleanor brought Christmas cards and her mother's address book and they wrote cards together. The following year they talked through each card, but Eleanor had to write the holiday message; her mother could still copy an address with prompting. The third Christmas Eleanor's mother no longer remembered most of the people, but still enjoyed listening to Eleanor talk about each card; that year her mother put the stamps on the envelopes.*

**Do reminiscence activities together.** As people's memories grow worse, they are able to remember less and less of recent events. Thus it makes sense to concentrate activities and conversation on events of long ago that are often remembered better and may be more pleasant. Making and labeling photo collages or albums together, taping or writing down old stories and memories, looking at books that trigger old memories can be therapeutic and enjoyable joint activities.

**Bring pets to visit.** For some people, pets are a great pleasure. More and more residences are beginning to have live-in pets, but bringing a friendly family pet to visit is also a good activity.

**Do grooming activities.** Give your relative a manicure, a gentle massage, a shave, particularly if these are difficult for staff to accomplish.

**Go for walks together.**

**Clean drawers** and closets together.

# COMMON EMOTIONAL REACTIONS OF FAMILIES

Making the decision to move your relative to a care residence is likely to be an emotional and confusing time despite your thorough planning and the advice given to you. It may help you to understand that your reactions to the decision and to the actual move are very common and natural.

**Guilt.** At the top of the list and many times the strongest emotion is guilt. Feeling guilty is often related to feeling that you "should" be able to continue caring for your relative at home. You may feel that you aren't fulfilling your responsibility despite having cared for your relative a long time. Or you may feel guilty because of a promise not to move your relative to a care residence.

*If you are feeling guilty, it may help to think about what you are giving your relative.*

- If you are feeling guilty about moving your relative, it may help you to think about what you are giving your relative: an opportunity to be with other residents and staff in a safe place where you can visit and not be distracted by caregiving responsibilities.

- It can help to say, "I moved my mother", rather than "I put (or placed) my mother in a residence."

- Guilt usually lessens when both you and your relative become more comfortable with the new home, staff, and schedule.

*Carl was totally opposed to moving his wife, but following his heart attack their daughter insisted. The first few weeks following the move, he was consumed by guilt. But much to his surprise, Carl found that his relationship with his wife improved. Although she still asked to go home occasionally, she enjoyed the activities and companionship of other residents. She was no longer angry at Carl all the time, because he was not the one who was "forcing" her to bathe and change clothes. His guilt quickly lessened as he realized that his wife was adjusting well.*

**Uncertainty and anxiety.** A common question caregivers often ask themselves is, "Am I doing the right thing?" There are many factors that can lead to feelings of uneasiness: cost, how and when your relative adapts to her new home, differences in the way the staff care for your relative. If you find you are questioning your decision to move your relative, you are not alone. Feeling lost and uncertain about the decision and the future is natural.

- Recognize that anxiety is a common reaction to uncertainty. You don't know if moving will be better for you and your relative because neither of you has experienced it yet. Often families have to get through the experience of moving and the adjustment period before they feel confident in their decision. There are adjustments throughout the moving process. When you feel more certain and secure about the move, anxiety will likely decrease.

- Talk openly about how you are feeling with people who have supported you through the illness: friends, family, pastor or rabbi or other caregivers.

- Families often feel especially ambivalent when they do not feel supported by other family members or friends. If there is conflict within your family about the moving decision, it may be helpful to schedule a family meeting. A professional such as a social worker, nurse, doctor, pastor, or counselor can function as an outside mediator and help you and your family talk about feelings and plans for care.

*Talk openly about how you are feeling with people who have supported you through the illness.*

*Alice's aunt kept saying to her, "How can you move Marie, my little sister, into a facility? I can't believe you are doing this to your mother!" This continuous criticism increased Alice's anxiety, guilt, and uncertainty. Finally she asked her aunt to meet with her and the social worker at the home care agency. The social worker was able to help Alice's aunt understand how unsafe and isolated Marie was at home. Together they reviewed different options for her care. Eventually Alice's aunt was able to agree with the need for a move and helped to choose the new residence.*

If you are feeling anxious in reaction to your relative's anxiety after the move,

- Talk to the appropriate staff person about your relative's adjustment and needs.

- Let the staff know about specific measures that you found successful in reducing your relative's anxiety.

- Try to understand that your anxiety may be in response to your relative's anxiety.

- Ask the appropriate staff member when your relative is most and least anxious. Sometimes a new resident acts in new or strange ways during family visiting and not during other parts of the day.

*Ann was terribly concerned because her husband was so distressed whenever she visited during the first three weeks after the move. He would beg to go home, get angry, try to follow her out the door, and generally make her visits a misery. Finally she met with the resident care coordinator about her concerns. Ann discovered that most of the time, her husband reserved his anxiety and anger for her visits; when she was not present, he was relatively content and involved. Staff began keeping notes of his activities and comments on each shift, so that Ann could be aware of his adjustment process when she was not present. They also gave her some suggestions for handling his outbursts when she visited, and they helped distract him when it was time for her to leave. After a few more weeks, most of his anger and anxiety subsided during her visits.*

**Grief.** You may find that the move into residential care intensifies feelings of grief, especially sadness and anger. Grieving is a natural reaction to the loss of a relative's abilities and the changing roles for you, the caregiver.

- It is better to feel the sadness or anger than to fight it. You may find it helpful to talk about the losses with your family members, a counselor, or with other caregivers in a support group.

- If you feel more comfortable expressing your sadness privately, set aside some time to do this.

- Try to schedule one enjoyable non-caregiving activity each day following the move. Feelings of grief usually lessen with time.

*After her mother moved to residential care, Becky felt angry and sad much of the time. In talking to a fellow caregiver, Becky realized she was angry at the disease at the same time she felt sad that her mother needed more care than she could give.*

**Failure.** If you are the kind of person who is used to solving all problems and making things better, you may be feeling like a failure because you moved your relative into a care residence. It may help to know that many caregivers feel they did not try hard enough when, in fact, a great amount of love, time, and energy was dedicated to caring for their relative.

- If you have kept a diary or a journal, take some time to read it. Sometimes all the things that caregivers have done are forgotten with the passage of time. A diary often is a good reminder. Tell yourself you did everything you could have done.

- Think about all the changes you experienced over time, all the challenges you took on and the problems you were able to solve.

- Congratulate yourself for being flexible, caring, and hard working. No one can make this disease go away.

**Fatigue.** Caring for a person with dementia often requires an enormous amount of physical and emotional energy. This may be the reason that you moved your relative. Making the decision and then the actual move also can deplete your energy.

*Grieving is a natural reaction to the loss of a relative's abilities and the changing roles for you, the caregiver.*

Caregivers are often unaware of why they may feel more tired at this time.

- Try to recognize that you may not have the energy to do all the things you normally do. It takes time to recover emotionally and physically from moving a loved one to residential care.

- Decide what tasks are necessary to do, what tasks you would like to do, and what tasks can wait until later. Begin doing the things on the "Must Do" list. Praise yourself for your accomplishments.

- Get adequate rest and sleep.

**Relief.** Relief may or may not be the expected reaction after a relative has moved. You may feel enormous relief that others are involved in the care and supervision of your loved one. Or you may not feel relieved at all because it is difficult to share the care with other caregivers. Or you may feel relief quickly followed by guilt.

- It is important to realize that these feelings are normal and common.

- Relief may be delayed until you and your relative have adjusted to the move.

- Try to remember that adjustment to moving takes time for everyone.

*The Ward family was very relieved to see their father move to assisted living. His wife had not been an adequate caregiver, and she was not fond of his kids, besides. However, George Ward gave the staff and his family a very difficult time for several months. Frequently, he called his wife and kids in the middle of the night, continually paced the halls throughout the day, and refused to bathe or shave. The staff and family worked with George's doctor on medications for anxiety and depression, held a number of care plan meetings, and were beginning to think this move would not work, when finally he calmed down. It had taken three months, but when George finally adjusted, he made friends and became a favorite of staff.*

# COMMON EMOTIONAL REACTIONS OF NEW RESIDENTS

Some of the more common reactions to moving are briefly discussed here. Keep in mind, however, that there are great individual differences among people with dementia. Some people will experience many of these feelings; others may exhibit very few. Some will be traumatized by the move; others will adjust easily.

**Grief.** Any move that is not voluntary will be perceived as a loss. In fact, it is a series of losses – loss of the ability to make one's own decisions, loss of the familiar environment and routine, some loss of autonomy. Under the circumstances, it is normal and expected for someone to feel grief, although this may show up in unexpected ways in people with dementia. Most of the reactions listed below may well be part of your relative's grieving process.

**Confusion and disorientation.** All of us feel a little confused and disoriented after we move to a new place. This is much more pronounced in people with dementia, because they have less ability to remember where they are. Usually this will improve as they adjust.

*A* good approach is to help the person learn her way around. Practice walking to the dining room or the courtyard. Point out landmarks along the way and identify characteristics of your relative's room such as "This is your room. The one with the flowers beside the door." Doing this during every visit may help reduce your relative's confusion and disorientation during the initial days after the move.

*A* If your relative has moved following an illness or hospitalization, you may see much more disorientation and confusion than before the illness. Be aware that it is common for individuals with dementia to decline somewhat following an illness; this may be either temporary or permanent.

**Anxiety and agitation.** Increased anxiety often accompanies increased confusion. Routines, familiar

> *A*ll of us feel a little confused and disoriented after we move to a new place.

landscape, including people, have all been changed by the move. Again, most of us feel anxious after a big change – this may be more pronounced, particularly if your relative is someone who tends to be anxious anyway. Initially, your relative may be more anxious when you are there because she is uncertain of what she is expected to do.

- The first thing to recognize is that increased agitation and anxiety during the initial days and weeks following a move are common. Anxiety usually decreases as a person becomes more adjusted to her new surroundings, staff and routine.

- Try to remain calm when your relative is anxious. Reassure her that she is safe and you know where she is.

- If you are anxious about your relative's behavior, talk to the appropriate staff member about measures that might be taken to reduce the anxiety and agitation that your relative is experiencing.

- Think about what reassures your relative and brings her comfort. Give staff the words to use that might help, such as, "Fred, your son, is so glad you are here with us." One daughter found a picture frame that could have a short message taped into it. When her mother was anxious, staff would hand her the framed photo of her daughter. When the button was pushed, her daughter's voice said, "Mama, this is Alice. I am so glad you are safe. I will visit you soon."

- It is common for a new resident to state, "I want to go home" during the days and weeks following a move. It is natural to want to grant this wish, but not always in the resident's best interest. A visit home may increase agitation and set back adjustment during the initial weeks after a move. Check with the appropriate staff member about her views on taking your relative home for a visit or on an outing.

*It is common for a new resident to state, "I want to go home" during the days and weeks following a move.*

**Anger.** Anger is a very normal reaction to a move, especially when it is against a person's will or without her prior knowledge. As hard as it is for family members to handle, it is to be expected. Sometimes people express their anger by complaining about the food, the staff, their room

43

or other residents. Sometimes a person directly expresses the anger at the family, making for uncomfortable visits and feelings of guilt.

- Generally, listening to the person and allowing her to express the anger is the best thing to do. If it becomes too difficult to listen, try changing the subject or involving her in an activity. If all else fails, you may want to leave and call later to see how your relative is doing.

- Acknowledge that you understand how she is feeling. Saying, "I am sorry you are feeling this way" may be helpful.

- Try not to argue the merits of living there or talk her out of her anger. This doesn't usually work!

**Denial.** It is common for people with dementia to deny that they have moved to this new home. "I don't live here!" is often said during the first few days and weeks. Sometimes it is simply memory loss. But it may also be part of the grieving process. Denial can be one of the hardest things which families and staff have to address.

- Trying to argue her into acceptance of her new home rarely works. It probably won't help to insist that this is her home. Try agreeing with her, sympathizing with her, or distracting her. "I know this is really hard for you," demonstrates to her that you are listening.

- Sometimes involving her in an activity or another conversation may work.

- If she becomes angry and intent on going to her "real home," ask for some help from a staff member. It may be better for you to leave at this point rather than continue to be upset by her denial.

- Denial often fades as a person adjusts to her new surroundings. But some residents never accept the fact of their new living situation. In these cases, families and staff learn to adjust their own expectations and reactions.

**Fatigue.** You can expect your relative to be more tired than usual. A change as major as moving is exhausting, and it may take all of her reserves to cope and gradually adjust to the new environment. It is not unusual for a new resident to sleep longer

*A change as major as moving is exhausting, and it may take all of her reserves to cope and gradually adjust to the new environment.*

at night or take more than the usual number of cat naps during the day to restore expended energy.

- Try not to push her past her limits.

- Short visits may be better than long ones. A quiet visit of sitting, having a snack together, or talking may be better than doing something more active.

**Withdrawal and sadness.** Don't be surprised if your relative is more withdrawn than usual. This is a common reaction to feeling sad or overwhelmed by the newness of everything.

- Talk to a staff member about the changes you are seeing. Ask her if the changes your relative is experiencing are within the normal range.

**Lost or sense of not belonging.** Your relative may complain about feeling lost, not having anything to do, or not knowing anyone. Feeling comfortable attending activities and being with other residents can take longer than you expect. Sometimes a new resident must adjust to being in the new environment before she can be comfortable in social situations.

- Ask a staff member if her attendance in activities and interactions with other residents is normal considering how long she has lived there.

- Discuss activities she might be interested in and ways staff might involve her in these activities.

- Often families feel so much guilt or are so anxious for their relative to be happy in her new home that they try to talk her out of feelings of anger, sadness, or denial.

- One of the hardest things for family members is to allow their relative to experience some of these feelings. The most important thing you can do is listen, acknowledge the feelings, and give your relative time to adjust and feel comfortable in her new home. Saying, "I can see that you are feeling sad," and holding her hand may bring some comfort.

- It is normal, and perhaps necessary, for people to experience some of these more difficult emotions. They are not unlike the feelings you may be experiencing. However, there can be positive feelings as well.

> *The most important thing you can do is listen, acknowledge the feelings, and give your relative time to adjust and feel comfortable in her new home.*

**Relief.** It is quite common for people with dementia to feel relieved when they move. Often they have felt that they have become a burden to their caregiver. Or they have begun to feel unsafe or bored in their old environment. For some people, there is great security in having people around and a routine to follow.

**Excitement.** Sometimes our relatives surprise us with a totally different reaction than we expect. Occasionally new residents are excited by their new environment. Those who have been living alone or with a single relative may be overwhelmed by the number of people and things to do, but also excited by them.

# WORKSHEET

Worksheet for

# Choosing a Residential Care Setting:
## Things to Look for, Questions to Ask

*Moving a Relative with Memory Loss*, Whisp Publications, © 2006 www.whisppub.com

Name of residence _____ Date of visit _____

Type of facility:  ☐ small group home      ☐ specialized memory care

☐ assisted living      ☐ nursing home

Address _____ Phone _____

Contact person _____

## LICENSING

State licensing requirements vary; some types of residential care in some states do not require licenses.

|  | Yes | No | Comments |
|---|---|---|---|
| *Facility licensed by the state* | ☐ | ☐ | |
| *Most recent inspection report reviewed.* | ☐ | ☐ | |

## THE ENVIRONMENT

|  | Yes | No | Comments |
|---|---|---|---|
| *Feels calm, comfortable & friendly* | ☐ | ☐ | |
| *Unpleasant odors* | ☐ | ☐ | |
| *Clean* | ☐ | ☐ | |
| *Well lighted* | ☐ | ☐ | |
| *Walking space indoors and outdoors* | ☐ | ☐ | |
| *Cues to help residents find the bathroom, bedroom, etc* | ☐ | ☐ | |
| *Private areas for family visiting* | ☐ | ☐ | |

## COST

*Monthly rate:* $_____

*Services included in the monthly rate*

*Services not included in the monthly rate*

*If there are levels of care, what is the process of determining when a resident needs the next level of care?*

| | Yes | No | Comments |
|---|---|---|---|
| *Accepts Medicaid* | ☐ | ☐ | |
| *Accepts long term care insurance* | ☐ | ☐ | |

## PERSONAL PRIVATE SPACE

Ask to see one or two residents' rooms.

| | Yes | No | Comments |
|---|---|---|---|
| *Allowed to bring personal possessions* | ☐ | ☐ | |
| *Clean and tidy* | ☐ | ☐ | |
| *Shared rooms: adequate space, enough privacy* | ☐ | ☐ | |

## RESIDENTS' APPEARANCE

It is important to realize that there may be reasons why some residents are not dressed when you visit – late start to their day, waiting for a bath, etc.

| | Yes | No | Comments |
|---|---|---|---|
| *Residents look neat, well groomed and clean.* | ☐ | ☐ | |
| *Residents appear to be odor free.* | ☐ | ☐ | |

## RESIDENTS' ABILITIES

Keep in mind that resident populations change constantly due to residents moving in and moving out.

| | Yes | No | Comments |
|---|---|---|---|
| *Residents appear to have similar abilities as my relative.* | ☐ | ☐ | |
| *I think my relative would be comfortable with the other residents.* | ☐ | ☐ | |

## INTERACTIONS BETWEEN STAFF AND RESIDENTS

| | Yes | No | Comments |
|---|---|---|---|
| *Staff speak respectfully to residents.* | ☐ | ☐ | |
| *Staff interact with residents.* | ☐ | ☐ | |
| *Staff are responsive to residents' needs.* | ☐ | ☐ | |

# ACTIVITIES

Ask to see the activity calendar and whether you can observe an activity.

| | Yes | No | Comments |
|---|---|---|---|
| *Many different types of activities are offered.* | ☐ | ☐ | |
| *There are activities that might interest and involve my relative.* | ☐ | ☐ | |
| *Activities are offered throughout the day.* | ☐ | ☐ | |

# STAFFING

| | # of staff | # of residents | Comments |
|---|---|---|---|
| Day shift | | | |
| Afternoon shift | | | |
| Night shift | | | |

| | Yes | No | Comments |
|---|---|---|---|
| *The staff to resident ratio includes direct care staff only.* | ☐ | ☐ | |

# STAFF TRAINING

| | Yes | No | Comments |
|---|---|---|---|
| *All staff are trained in dementia care.* | ☐ | ☐ | |
| *Staff training programs are scheduled regularly.* | ☐ | ☐ | |
| *Family members can attend training sessions.* | ☐ | ☐ | |

# MEDICAL CARE

| | Yes | No | Comments |
|---|---|---|---|
| *My relative's doctor can treat her here.* | ☐ | ☐ | |
| *Nurses are on staff. If yes, when?* | ☐ | ☐ | |

| | Available: | Not available: |
|---|---|---|
| *Types of medical care:* | | |

*Title and credentials of personnel who monitor and give medications:*

*The procedure for notifying families when there is a change in a resident's medical condition or behavior:*

## RESIDENT SELECTION

| | Yes | No | Comments |
|---|---|---|---|
| *Assessment fee* | ☐ | ☐ | |
| *Amount: $_____* | | | |
| *Refundable?* | ☐ | ☐ | |
| *What medical conditions are not accepted?* | | | |

*Assessment procedure: What medical records and tests are required before a person can move in?*

## RESIDENT DISCHARGE

*Medical conditions or behaviors that might cause a resident to be asked to leave:*

*Amount of notice given to families if a resident is asked to leave:*

## CARE PLAN

A care plan is a document that identifies a resident's needs and how her needs will be met. A resident's physical, spiritual, emotional, and recreational needs are addressed in a care plan that is discussed at a care conference.

| | Yes | No | Comments |
|---|---|---|---|
| *There is a care plan for each resident.* | ☐ | ☐ | |
| *Families are invited to care conferences.* | ☐ | ☐ | |

## FAMILY PROGRAMS AND SUPPORT

| | Yes | No | Comments |
|---|---|---|---|
| *Family support group* | ☐ | ☐ | |
| *Family education programs* | ☐ | ☐ | |
| *Family social events* | ☐ | ☐ | |

## END OF LIFE CARE

In some states legal documents are required to make end of life decisions for another person. This document may be called a living will or an advanced health care directive.

*Required documents to make end of life decisions for my relative:*

| | Yes | No | Comments |
|---|---|---|---|
| *Hospice care provided* | ☐ | ☐ | |

# SUGGESTED
# READINGS

# SUGGESTED READINGS

## For families caring for a relative with Alzheimer's disease:

Sherry M. Bell, *Visiting Mom: An Unexpected Gift.* Elder Press, 2000. A daughter shares how she learned to communicate and visit successfully with her mother in a nursing home.

Virginia Bell and David Troxel, *The Best Friends Approach to Alzheimer's Care.* Health Professions Press, 1997. Excellent overview of dementia for families; easy to read and excellent philosophical approach.

Virginia Bell and David Troxel, *A Dignified Life: The Best Friends' Approach to Alzheimer's Care, A Guide for Families.* Health Professions Press, 2002. Similar to above title; written specifically for families.

Robert Butler and Joanne Koenig Coste, *Learning to Speak Alzheimer's: A Groundbreaking Approach for Everyone Dealing with the Disease.* Houghton Mifflin Co., 2003. A wife uses her personal experience of caring for her husband to offer hundreds of practical tips to caregivers.

Nancy Mace and Peter Rabins, *The 36 Hour Day.* Johns Hopkins Press, 1991. Considered "The Bible" of Alzheimer's care. An excellent overall reference book.

Anne Robinson, Beth Spencer, Laurie White, *Understanding Difficult Behaviors: Some Practical Suggestions for Coping with Alzheimer's Disease and Related Illnesses.* Eastern Michigan University, 1989. Looks at a number of challenging behaviors, including wandering, incontinence, agitation, bathing. Discusses possible reasons for behaviors and lists strategies for dealing with them.

## For the person with Alzheimer's disease:

Helen Davies and Michael Jensen, *Alzheimer's: The Answers You Need.* Elder Books, 1998. Commonly asked questions and answers in an easy-to-read format.

## Memoirs written by individuals diagnosed with Alzheimer's disease:

Robert Davis, *My Journey into Alzheimer's.* Tyndale House, 1989. A minister in the early stages of Alzheimer's writes about his life and his experience with his illness.

Cary Smith Henderson, *Partial View: An Alzheimer's Journal.* Southern Methodist University Press, 1998. A professor dictates his experiences with dementia. Excerpts of his reflections are accompanied by photographs of him.

Lisa Snyder, Editor, *Speaking Our Minds: Personal Reflections from Individuals with Alzheimer's.* W.H. Freeman and Company, 1999. A social worker excerpts interviews with individuals with Alzheimer's disease, giving background information and her insightful reflections.

Made in the USA
Lexington, KY
05 February 2012